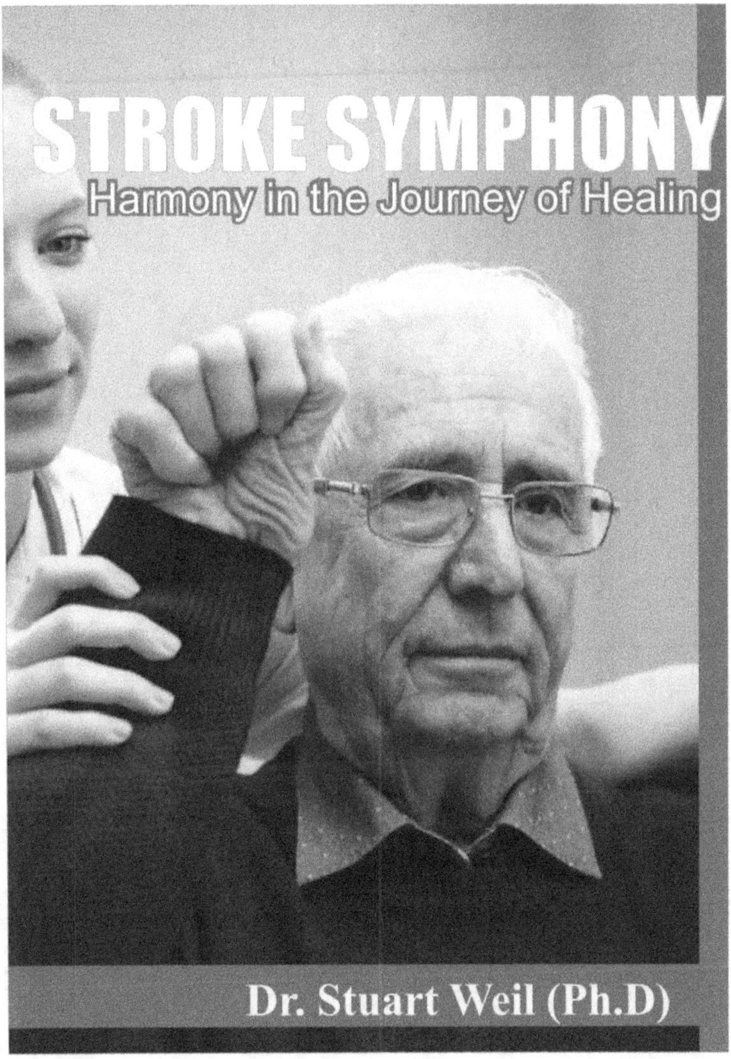

STROKE SYMPHONY
Harmony in the Journey of Healing

Dr. Stuart Weil (Ph.D)

this page is intentionally left blank

Dr. Stuart Weil

STROKE SYMPHONY
Harmony in the Journey of Healing

Dedication

I dedicate this book to all those who have supported me throughout *my days of intense agony in back ache.*

My wife, Gabriella,

my family,

my healthcare advisors,

able consultants, and nurses in the wards.

Without their care and support, it would have been a futile effort trying to put together this piece.

Table of Contents

Preface

In the realm of life's unexpected twists, the journey of stroke recovery stands as a testament to the indomitable spirit of the human soul. This guide is not just a collection of pages; it's a lifeline, a compass, and a companion for those navigating the uncharted territory of life after a stroke.

To the stroke survivors who have faced the storm and emerged on the other side, and to the caregivers who stand as pillars of strength, this book is a dedicated space for understanding, learning, and healing. It is an acknowledgment of the Challenges you've faced, a celebration of the victories you've achieved, and a roadmap for the journey that lies ahead.

As we step into this exploration of resilience, adaptation, and triumph, let us be united by a common thread—the unwavering belief that recovery is not just a destination but a continuous, evolving process. The stories within these pages are not just narratives; they are shared experiences that bind us together as a community of strength.

From the intricacies of rehabilitation to the profound impact on daily lives, we embark on a journey that delves into the heart of stroke recovery. Here, knowledge meets compassion, and every page is a step forward in understanding, supporting, and ultimately thriving in the face of adversity.

So, dear reader, fasten your seatbelt for a journey that goes beyond information—it's a journey of empowerment, connection, and the profound realization that, even in the face of a storm, there is resilience within that can weather any Challenge.

Welcome to a guide that transcends the ordinary—a guide for the brave, the hopeful, and those ready to embrace the path of resilience. The journey begins here.

There is life—and hope—after stroke. With time, new routines will become second nature. Rehabilitation can build your strength, capability and confidence. It can help you continue your daily activities despite the effects of your stroke.

If you are the caregiver, family member or friend of a stroke survivor, your role is vital. You should know the prevention plan and help your loved one to comply with the plan. With a committed health care team and a rehabilitation plan specific to their needs, most stroke survivors can prevent another stroke and thrive.

Welcome to a guide that transcends the ordinary—a guide for the brave, the hopeful, and those ready to embrace the path of resilience. The journey begins here.

CHAPTER ONE

ABOUT STROKE
What's Stroke?

Stroke is an event that affects the arteries of the brain. A stroke occurs when a blood vessel bringing blood to the brain gets blocked or ruptures (bursts). This means that the area of the brain the blocked or ruptured blood vessel supplies can't get the oxygen and nutrients it needs. Without oxygen, nerve cells can't function. Your brain controls your ability to move, feel, think and behave. Brain injury from a stroke may affect any of these functions. Several factors affect the ways people experience a stroke. They include:

1. Ischaemic Stroke
2. Haemorrhagic Stroke
3. Transient Ischaemic Attack

Ischemic stroke: occurs when a clot blocks a vessel supplying blood to the brain. The artery becomes narrowed or clogged, cutting off blood flow to brain cells. Ischemic strokes are the most common type of stroke.

Haemorrhagic stroke: happens when a blood vessel bursts (ruptures) in the brain. This type of stroke may affect large arteries in the brain or the small blood vessels deep within the brain. The rupture keeps the surrounding areas of the brain from getting needed oxygen. Haemorrhagic strokes are less common than ischemic strokes.

Transient ischemic attacks (TIAs): are often called "warning strokes." TIAs produce symptoms just like stroke, but typically last a shorter amount of time. They don't usually cause lasting damage. But they are major predictors of future stroke. If you suspect you've had or are having a TIA, don't ignore it!

Call 9-1-1. Get immediate medical attention, even if the symptoms go away.

Common risk factors for strokes include high blood pressure, smoking, diabetes, high cholesterol, and a family history of strokes. Other factors such as age, gender, and ethnicity can also contribute.

Symptoms of a stroke can vary but often include sudden numbness or weakness in the face, arm, or leg, especially on one side of the body. Other signs may include confusion, trouble speaking or understanding speech, severe headache, dizziness, and difficulty walking.

The acronym **FAST** is often used to help people recognize and respond to the signs of a stroke:

F: Face Drooping
A: Arm Weakness
S: Speech Difficulty
T: Time to Call Emergency Services

Treatment for a stroke depends on the type and cause but often involves medication, surgery, or rehabilitation to help the survivor regain lost functions.

Stroke survivors may face various Challenges, and rehabilitation plays a crucial role in helping them regain independence and improve their quality of life. Post-stroke care may involve physical therapy, occupational therapy, and speech therapy, among other interventions. The extent of recovery can vary, and ongoing support from healthcare professionals, caregivers, and support groups is essential for stroke survivors.

EARLY TREATMENT
Early treatment of ischemic stroke Ischemic stroke happens when a blood clot blocks a vessel supplying blood to the brain. It's the most common type, accounting for 87% of all strokes. The treatment goal is to dissolve or remove the clot. To dissolve a clot, a medicine called alteplase (tPA) is given through an IV

(intravenous line). It works by dissolving the clot so blood can flow again. Alteplase can save lives and reduce the long-term effects of stroke. It needs to be given within three hours of the start of stroke symptoms (up to 4.5 hours for some eligible patients). To remove a clot involves a procedure called mechanical thrombectomy. Doctors use a wire-cage device called a stent retriever to remove a large blood clot. They thread a catheter through an artery in the groin up to the blocked artery in the brain. The stent opens and grabs the clot, allowing doctors to remove the stent with the trapped clot. Special suction tubes may also be used to remove the clot. This procedure must be done within up to six to 24 hours of stroke symptom onset and after the patient has received alteplase, if eligible. Patients must meet certain criteria to be eligible for this procedure.

Early treatment of haemorrhagic stroke
Haemorrhagic stroke happens when a blood vessel bursts (ruptures) and bleeds within or around the brain. Blood vessels can become

weak due to a ballooning of part of the vessel (aneurysm). Other times there may be a tangle of blood vessels within the brain that didn't form normally, making them weak (arteriovenous malformation or AVM). When high blood pressure isn't controlled, it puts strain on weakened blood vessels that can lead to the ruptures that cause stroke. The treatment goal is to stop the bleeding. For some patients, a small tube (catheter) with a camera is threaded through a major artery in an arm or leg and guided to the area of the bleed in the brain. The camera gives the surgeon a detailed view of the area to help fix the problem. Once the catheter is guided to the source of the bleeding, it leaves a mechanism, such as a coil, to prevent further rupture. This type of procedure is less invasive than standard surgical treatment. Sometimes surgery is required to secure a blood vessel at the base of the aneurysm.

Common Changes After a Stroke

Stroke can lead to a variety of changes in a person's life, impacting different aspects such as physical abilities, communication skills, cognitive functions, emotional well-being, and even personality. It's important to note that the extent and nature of these changes can vary widely among individuals. Here are common changes observed after a stroke:

CHAPTER TWO

After a Stroke

Stroke can lead to a variety of changes in a person's life, impacting different aspects such as physical abilities, communication skills, cognitive functions, emotional well-being, and even personality. It's important to note that the extent and nature of these changes can vary widely among individuals. Here are common changes observed after a stroke:

Physical Changes

Weakness or Paralysis: Depending on the location and severity of the stroke, there may be weakness or paralysis in one side of the body.

Coordination Issues: Stroke survivors may experience difficulties with balance and coordination.

Mobility Challenges: Walking and other motor skills may be affected, leading to changes in the ability to move independently.

Communication Changes:

Aphasia: A common language impairment, aphasia can affect speaking, understanding, reading, and writing.

Dysarthria: This condition results in difficulty with articulation and control of the muscles used in speech.

Cognitive Changes:

Memory Impairment: Short-term or long-term memory may be affected, impacting daily activities and routines.

Attention and Concentration: Stroke survivors may experience difficulties in focusing attention and maintaining concentration.

Executive Functioning: Challenges in planning, organizing, problem-solving, and decision-making may arise.

Emotional Changes:

Depression: It's not uncommon for stroke survivors to experience feelings of sadness or depression, which may be linked to the physical and emotional Challenges they face.

Anxiety: Concerns about the future, fear of another stroke, or changes in social roles can contribute to anxiety.

Mood Swings: Emotional lability, characterized by rapid mood swings, may occur.

Personality Changes:

Emotional Expression: Some stroke survivors may exhibit changes in emotional expression, such as inappropriate laughter or crying.

Disinhibition: There could be a lack of impulse control or changes in social behaviour.

Sensory Changes:

Vision Impairment: Visual disturbances or partial blindness may occur.

Sensory Loss: Changes in the sense of touch or proprioception (awareness of body position) can be experienced.

Swallowing Difficulties:

Dysphagia: Stroke survivors may have difficulty swallowing, leading to Challenges with eating and drinking.

Fatigue:

Physical and Mental Fatigue: Stroke survivors often experience fatigue, both physical and mental, which can impact daily activities.

Social and Vocational Impact:

Social Isolation: Changes in communication, mobility, and energy levels can contribute to social isolation.

Occupational Challenges: Returning to work or engaging in previous activities may be challenging.

Sleep Disturbances:

Insomnia or Hypersomnia: Sleep patterns may be disrupted, leading to difficulties in falling asleep or staying awake during the day.

Pain:

Post-Stroke Pain: Some survivors may experience pain, including headaches or pain in the affected limbs.

Changes in Self-Perception:

Loss of Identity: Coping with the changes brought about by a stroke can lead to shifts in self-perception and self-esteem.

It's important to recognize that stroke recovery is a complex and individualized process. Rehabilitation strategies are often tailored to address the specific Challenges faced by each stroke survivor. Regular follow-up with healthcare professionals, including neurologists, physiatrists, and therapists, is crucial to monitor progress and adjust interventions accordingly. Additionally, ongoing support from caregivers, support groups, and mental health professionals is vital for the holistic well-being of stroke survivors.

Rehabilitation, including physical therapy, occupational therapy, and speech therapy, plays a crucial role in helping stroke survivors regain functional abilities and adapt to these changes. Additionally, emotional support from healthcare professionals, family, and friends is essential in the recovery process. Each individual's journey is unique, and a personalized approach to rehabilitation and support is crucial for optimizing outcomes.

CHAPTER THREE

Rehabilitation

Rehabilitation after a stroke is a critical and comprehensive process aimed at helping stroke survivors regain functional abilities, independence, and quality of life. It involves a multidisciplinary approach and typically includes physical therapy, occupational therapy, speech-language therapy, and, in some cases, psychological support. The importance of rehabilitation in stroke recovery is multifaceted:

Restoring Functionality:

Physical Therapy: Helps improve mobility, strength, and coordination. Exercises are tailored to address specific motor impairments caused by the stroke.

Occupational Therapy: Focuses on daily living skills, such as dressing, eating, and bathing, to enhance independence.

Addressing Communication Challenges:

Speech-Language Therapy: Aims to improve communication skills, including speaking, understanding, reading, and writing. It also addresses swallowing difficulties (dysphagia).

Cognitive Rehabilitation:

Cognitive Therapy: Targets cognitive impairments, such as memory loss, attention deficits, and executive function Challenges.

Emotional Support:

Psychological Counselling: Helps stroke survivors cope with emotional Challenges, such as depression, anxiety, and adjustment to life changes.

Preventing Complications:

Preventing Secondary Complications: Rehabilitation helps minimize the risk of secondary issues such as muscle atrophy, joint contractures, and pressure sores.

Enhancing Social Integration:

Social Work and Support Groups: Address the social and emotional aspects of stroke recovery, promoting social interaction and reducing feelings of isolation.

Caregiver Training:

Education and Training: Rehabilitation involves educating caregivers on how to assist with daily activities, provide emotional support, and ensure a safe home environment.

Maximizing Independence:

Functional Independence: Rehabilitation aims to maximize a stroke survivor's ability to perform daily activities independently.

Adapting to Changes:

Adaptive Strategies: Therapists work with stroke survivors and caregivers to develop adaptive strategies for dealing with residual Challenges.

Role of the Caregiver:

Support and Encouragement:
Caregivers play a crucial role in providing emotional support, encouragement, and motivation during the recovery process.

Assistance with Activities of Daily Living (ADLs):

Caregivers help with daily tasks such as bathing, dressing, grooming, and meal preparation, especially if the stroke survivor has physical limitations.

Medication Management:
Caregivers may assist in managing medications, ensuring that the stroke survivor follows prescribed treatment plans.

Communication Advocacy:
Caregivers can support communication therapy exercises and provide a supportive environment for the stroke survivor to practice communication skills.

Facilitating Rehabilitation Exercises:
Caregivers often play a role in supporting and encouraging the completion of prescribed rehabilitation exercises at home.

Advocacy and Coordination of Care:
Caregivers may serve as advocates, communicating with healthcare professionals, coordinating appointments, and ensuring the stroke survivor receives comprehensive care.

Role of Family:

Family involvement and support play a crucial role in the rehabilitation and overall well-being of a stroke patient. The extent of family involvement can significantly impact the patient's recovery and adjustment to life after a stroke. Here are several ways in which family involvement and support benefit a stroke patient:

Emotional Support:

Reducing Emotional Stress: A stroke can be emotionally challenging for the patient. Family support helps alleviate stress, anxiety, and depression by providing a stable and caring environment.

Coping with Emotional Changes: Families can assist the patient in coping with emotional changes, including mood swings and potential personality changes that may occur after a stroke.

Motivation and Encouragement:

Promoting Rehabilitation Motivation: Family members can motivate and encourage the patient to actively participate in rehabilitation exercises and therapy sessions, fostering a positive mindset and commitment to recovery.

Assistance with Daily Activities:

Aiding in Daily Tasks: Stroke survivors may experience Challenges with daily activities. Family members can provide assistance with tasks such as dressing, grooming, bathing, and meal preparation, promoting independence while ensuring safety.

Advocacy in Healthcare Settings:

Communication with Healthcare Professionals: Family members can serve as advocates for the patient, communicating with healthcare professionals, asking questions, and ensuring that the patient's needs and preferences are addressed in the care plan.

Monitoring Medications and Treatment Plans:

Medication Management: Family members can help ensure that the patient adheres to prescribed medications and follows treatment plans outlined by healthcare professionals.

Facilitating Communication:

Supporting Speech Therapy: If the stroke has affected communication skills, family members can support speech therapy exercises and engage in effective communication strategies to enhance understanding.

Creating a Supportive Home Environment:

Home Modifications: Family involvement may include making necessary home modifications to ensure a safe and accessible environment for the stroke survivor.

Social Engagement and Community Integration:

Organizing Social Activities: Family members can organize social activities and outings to help the patient reintegrate into the community, reducing feelings of isolation.

Financial and Legal Support:

Navigating Financial and Legal Matters: Family members can assist with financial and legal matters, including insurance claims, paperwork, and ensuring that necessary arrangements are in place.

Educating the Family:

Strengthening Caregiver Skills: Family members can undergo training to understand the specific needs of the stroke survivor, including rehabilitation exercises, assistive devices, and strategies for managing Challenges.

Providing Respite Care:

Preventing Caregiver Burnout: Family involvement includes recognizing the importance of respite care, allowing family caregivers to take breaks to prevent burnout and maintain their own well-being.

Celebrating Achievements:

Positive Reinforcement: Family members can celebrate the patient's achievements, no matter how small, providing positive reinforcement and motivation for continued progress.

Long-Term Planning:

Assistance with Long-Term Care Planning: In cases where the stroke has resulted in significant disability, family involvement is crucial in discussing and planning for long-term care needs.

Family involvement is most beneficial when it is collaborative, supportive, and aligned with the preferences and needs of the stroke patient. Regular communication, flexibility, and a holistic approach to care contribute to a positive rehabilitation experience and improved overall quality of life for the stroke survivor.

Role of Healthcare Professional:

Continued Monitoring and Adjustment:

- Rehabilitation is an ongoing process that requires regular monitoring and adjustment. The healthcare team, including therapists and physicians, will assess progress and make changes to the rehabilitation plan as needed.

Prevention of Recurrent Strokes:

- Education about lifestyle changes, medication management, and regular follow-up care are important aspects of rehabilitation aimed at preventing future strokes.

Community Reintegration:

- Rehabilitation often includes strategies to facilitate community reintegration, helping the stroke survivor participate in social activities and engage with the community.

Technology-Assisted Rehabilitation:

- Advancements in technology, such as virtual reality and robotics, are increasingly being used in stroke rehabilitation to enhance motor skills and improve outcomes.

Promoting Holistic Well-being:

- Rehabilitation addresses not only physical aspects but also the psychological and emotional well-being of the stroke survivor. It aims to improve overall quality of life.

Caregiver Self-Care:

- Recognizing the importance of caregiver well-being is crucial. Caregivers need to take care of their own physical and mental health to effectively support the stroke survivor.

Long-Term Care Planning:

- For some stroke survivors with severe disabilities, long-term care planning may be necessary. This could involve home modifications, adaptive equipment, and consideration of assisted living or nursing care facilities.

Patient and Caregiver Empowerment:

- Empowering both the stroke survivor and the caregiver with knowledge and skills is fundamental to successful rehabilitation. This includes understanding the condition, knowing how to manage Challenges, and setting realistic goals.

Role of the Patient:

The role of the stroke patient in the rehabilitation process is crucial for a successful recovery. While healthcare professionals and caregivers provide support and guidance, the active participation and commitment of the stroke survivor are fundamental. Here are key aspects of the stroke patient's role in rehabilitation:

1. **Active Participation:**
   Actively engage in rehabilitation exercises, therapy sessions, and prescribed activities. Consistent effort is important for maximizing recovery.

2. **Communication with Healthcare Team:**
   Communicate openly with healthcare professionals about experiences, concerns, and progress. Sharing information helps

tailor the rehabilitation plan to individual needs.

4. **Setting Realistic Goals:**
   Work collaboratively with the healthcare team to set realistic and achievable goals. Establish short-term and long-term objectives to measure progress.

5. **Adherence to Treatment Plans:**
   Adhere to prescribed medications, lifestyle changes, and therapeutic interventions. Compliance with the treatment plan is vital for optimal outcomes.

6. **Self-Advocacy:**
   Advocate for personal needs and preferences. Be an active participant in decisions regarding care, rehabilitation strategies, and long-term goals.

7. **Emotional Well-being:**
   Recognize and address emotional Challenges that may arise during recovery. Seek support when needed, and actively participate in strategies to improve emotional well-being.

8. **Home Exercises and Activities:**

Follow through with prescribed exercises and activities at home. Consistency in performing exercises enhances the effectiveness of rehabilitation.

9. **Lifestyle Modifications:**
    Embrace necessary lifestyle changes to reduce risk factors for stroke recurrence. This may include dietary adjustments, regular exercise, and smoking cessation.

10. **Patience and Persistence:**
    Understand that recovery is a gradual process, and improvements may take time. Patience and persistence are key elements in the rehabilitation journey.

11. **Feedback and Communication with Caregiver:**
    Communicate openly with the caregiver about needs, preferences, and any Challenges faced. Collaboration between the stroke survivor and caregiver is essential for effective support.

12. **Community Engagement:**
    Participate in community activities and social interactions as part of the rehabilitation process. Reintegrating into

the community can contribute to overall well-being.

13. **Education and Self-Management:**
Be proactive in learning about the stroke, its effects, and self-management strategies. Education empowers the stroke survivor to take an active role in their own care.

14. **Celebrating Milestones:**
Acknowledge and celebrate achievements and milestones, no matter how small. Recognizing progress can boost motivation and morale.

By actively participating in the rehabilitation process, stroke survivors contribute significantly to their own recovery and well-being. Open communication, commitment to prescribed interventions, and a positive mindset are essential elements in maximizing the potential for improvement and achieving a fulfilling post-stroke life.

CHAPTER FOUR

Tips For Elegantly Choosing A REHABILITATION Centre

Choosing the right rehabilitation facility is a crucial step in the recovery journey after a stroke or any other medical condition. Here are some tips to consider when selecting a rehabilitation facility:

1. **Assess the Rehabilitation Services Offered:**
   Ensure the facility provides a comprehensive range of rehabilitation services, including physical therapy, occupational therapy, speech-language therapy, and other specialized therapies that may be required based on the individual's needs.

2. **Evaluate the Expertise of the Rehabilitation Team:**
Research the qualifications and experience of the healthcare professionals at the facility, including therapists, nurses, and physicians. A skilled and experienced team is essential for effective rehabilitation.

3. **Consider Accreditation and Certification:**
Check if the rehabilitation facility is accredited and certified by relevant healthcare authorities. Accreditation ensures that the facility meets certain standards of quality and safety.

4. **Review Patient Outcomes and Success Stories:**
Look for information on patient outcomes and success stories. Testimonials from previous patients or their families can provide insights into the facility's effectiveness in rehabilitation.

5. **Accessibility and Location:**
Consider the location of the facility in relation to the patient's home and the

accessibility of the facility. Proximity to family and friends can be important for emotional support.

6. **Facility Amenities and Environment:**
Assess the overall environment and amenities of the facility. A clean, comfortable, and well-maintained environment can positively impact the rehabilitation experience.

7. **Availability of Specialized Programs:**
If the stroke survivor has specific needs, such as stroke-specific rehabilitation programs or programs for coexisting conditions, ensure that the facility offers these specialized services.

8. **Patient-Centred Approach:**
Look for a facility that adopts a patient-centred approach, involving the individual and their family in the development of the rehabilitation plan. Personalized care plans are more effective.

9. **Transition and Continuity of Care:**
Inquire about the facility's approach to transition and continuity of care. A seamless transition from acute care to

rehabilitation and a clear plan for post-rehabilitation support are important.

10. **Family Involvement and Support:**
Assess the level of involvement and support that the facility encourages from family members. Family participation is often crucial for the success of rehabilitation.

11. **Insurance Coverage and Financial Considerations:**
Verify the insurance coverage for rehabilitation services and understand the financial aspects of the program. Check if the facility accepts the individual's insurance plan.

12. **Visit the Facility and Ask Questions:**
Schedule a visit to the rehabilitation facility and ask questions about the programs, services, and staff. Observing the facility first-hand can provide valuable insights.

13. **References and Recommendations:**
Seek recommendations from healthcare professionals, primary care physicians, or

other individuals who have experience with rehabilitation facilities. Personal references can be valuable.

14. **Community Integration Programs:** Inquire about programs that facilitate community integration and social engagement. Community activities and support can contribute to a well-rounded rehabilitation experience.

Taking the time to carefully evaluate rehabilitation options can contribute to a more effective and positive recovery experience. It's important to choose a facility that aligns with the individual's specific needs and preferences.

CHAPTER FIVE

Proactive Strategies

Preventing another stroke is crucial for individuals who have experienced a stroke and is essential for maintaining overall health. Here are some detailed strategies for preventing another stroke, both at home and in the workplace:

Coping At Home:

1. Medication Adherence:

   Follow Prescribed Medications: Take medications exactly as prescribed by healthcare professionals. These may include blood thinners, antihypertensives, and cholesterol-lowering drugs.

2. Lifestyle Modifications:

Healthy Diet: Adopt a diet rich in fruits, vegetables, whole grains, lean proteins, and low-fat dairy. Limit salt, saturated fats, and trans fats.

Regular Exercise: Engage in regular physical activity, aiming for at least 150 minutes of moderate-intensity aerobic exercise per week, as recommended by healthcare professionals.

Maintain a Healthy Weight: Achieve and maintain a healthy weight to reduce the risk of hypertension, diabetes, and other cardiovascular risk factors.

3. Blood Pressure Management:

Regular Monitoring: Keep track of blood pressure regularly, and work with healthcare professionals to manage hypertension effectively.

4. Smoking Cessation:

Quit Smoking: If the individual smokes, quitting is essential. Smoking is a significant risk factor for stroke and other cardiovascular diseases.

5. Alcohol Moderation:
    Limit Alcohol Intake: If alcohol is consumed, do so in moderation. Excessive alcohol intake can contribute to hypertension and other health issues.

6. Regular Health Check-ups:
    Regular Check-ups: Schedule regular health check-ups with healthcare professionals to monitor blood pressure, cholesterol levels, and overall health.

7. Managing Diabetes:
    Control Blood Sugar: If diabetic, manage blood sugar levels through medication, diet, and lifestyle changes.

8. Home Safety:
    Fall Prevention: Minimize the risk of falls by removing tripping hazards,

installing grab bars in bathrooms, and using non-slip mats.

9. Stress Management:
    Practice Stress-Reduction Techniques: Engage in stress-reducing activities such as meditation, deep breathing exercises, or hobbies to manage stress levels.

Coping In the Workplace:

1. Workplace Ergonomics:
    Ergonomic Design: Ensure a well-designed workspace to promote good posture and reduce the risk of musculoskeletal issues that may contribute to stress and hypertension.

2. Regular Breaks and Movement:
    Take Breaks: Encourage regular breaks to stand, stretch, and move around, promoting circulation and reducing sedentary behaviour.

3. Healthy Eating Habits:

Access to Healthy Options: Provide access to healthy food options in workplace cafeterias or break areas. Encourage employees to make nutritious choices.

4. Physical Activity Programs:
Promote Exercise: Implement workplace wellness programs that encourage physical activity, such as walking Challenges or exercise classes.

5. Smoking Cessation Support:
Support Quitting: Offer resources and support for employees who want to quit smoking, such as smoking cessation programs or counselling.

6. Stress Reduction Programs:
Wellness Initiatives: Implement stress reduction programs, such as mindfulness sessions, yoga, or mental health resources, to support employees' overall well-being.

7. Health Screenings:

Regular Health Screenings: Provide opportunities for health screenings, including blood pressure checks and cholesterol screenings, to promote early detection and management of risk factors.

8. Flexible Work Arrangements:

Flexible Schedules: Consider offering flexible work arrangements to accommodate individual health needs and reduce stress.

It's important to note that preventing another stroke is a comprehensive and ongoing effort that involves both individual lifestyle choices and supportive environments. Workplaces can play a significant role in promoting employee health through wellness initiatives and creating an environment that supports healthy choices. Additionally, collaboration with healthcare professionals for regular monitoring and adjustments to the prevention plan is essential.

CHAPTER SIX

Signs and symptoms of Stroke

Recognizing the signs and symptoms of a stroke is crucial for early intervention and can contribute to stroke prevention. Understanding these signs allows individuals to seek prompt medical attention, potentially minimizing the impact of a stroke. The signs and symptoms of a stroke are often summarized by the acronym FAST, which stands for Face, Arms, Speech, and Time. Here's a breakdown:

Face:

Sign: Sudden drooping or numbness on one side of the face.

Relevance to Prevention: Facial drooping can be a sign of facial muscle weakness, indicating a disruption in blood supply to the brain. Recognizing this symptom early can prompt individuals to seek medical attention for preventive measures.

Arms:

Sign: Sudden weakness or numbness in one arm or both arms.

Relevance to Prevention: Arm weakness is often associated with motor function impairment caused by a stroke. Early recognition can lead to timely intervention and strategies for preventing future strokes.

Speech:

Sign: Sudden difficulty speaking, slurred speech, or an inability to articulate words.

Relevance to Prevention: Speech difficulties can indicate impairment in the language centres of the brain. Recognizing these symptoms early can prompt individuals to seek medical attention for preventive measures and risk factor management.

Time:

Sign: Time is critical in stroke. If any of the above signs are observed, it's essential to seek emergency medical attention immediately.

Relevance to Prevention: The sooner medical intervention occurs, the better the chances of preventing long-term damage and reducing the risk of subsequent strokes. Time is a critical factor in receiving appropriate medical care and treatment.

In addition to the **FAST** acronym, other symptoms and warning signs of a stroke may include:

Sudden severe headache: Unexplained and severe headaches, especially when accompanied by other symptoms, can be indicative of a stroke.

Trouble walking or loss of coordination: Sudden difficulty walking, dizziness, or loss of coordination may be signs of a stroke.

Awareness and Education: Understanding these signs and symptoms increase awareness about the urgency of seeking medical help. This awareness is crucial for stroke prevention, as early intervention can prevent further damage.

Risk Factor Management: Recognizing the signs allows individuals to be proactive in managing stroke risk factors. Lifestyle changes, medication adherence, and regular medical check-ups can help prevent the occurrence of a stroke.

It's important for individuals to be familiar with these signs and symptoms, not only to respond promptly in case of a stroke but also to take preventive measures. Managing risk factors such as hypertension, diabetes, high cholesterol, and adopting a healthy lifestyle can significantly reduce the likelihood of experiencing a stroke. Regular medical check-ups and discussions with healthcare professionals about individual risk factors are essential components of stroke prevention.

In addition to recognizing the signs and symptoms of a stroke and actively managing risk factors, there are several more preventive measures and lifestyle changes that individual can adopt to reduce their risk of stroke:

Lifestyle Modifications:

Healthy Diet:

Adopt a diet rich in fruits, vegetables, whole grains, lean proteins, and low-fat dairy. The Dietary Approaches to Stop Hypertension (DASH) diet is often recommended for its emphasis on reducing sodium intake and promoting heart health.

Regular Physical Activity:

Engage in regular aerobic exercise, such as brisk walking, jogging, cycling, or swimming.

Aim for at least 150 minutes of moderate-intensity exercise per week.

Maintain a Healthy Weight:
Achieve and maintain a healthy weight through a combination of balanced diet and regular physical activity.

Limit Alcohol Intake:
If alcohol is consumed, do so in moderation. Excessive alcohol intake can raise blood pressure and contribute to stroke risk.

Quit Smoking:
Smoking is a major risk factor for stroke. Quitting smoking is one of the most effective ways to reduce the risk.

Manage Stress:
Practice stress-reducing techniques such as mindfulness, meditation, yoga, or hobbies that promote relaxation.

Medical Management:

Blood Pressure Control:

Regularly monitor blood pressure and work with healthcare professionals to maintain optimal levels. Hypertension is a significant risk factor for stroke.

Diabetes Management:

If diabetic, manage blood sugar levels through medication, diet, and lifestyle changes.

Cholesterol Management:

Control cholesterol levels through a combination of medication and lifestyle modifications.

Antiplatelet Medication:

In some cases, healthcare professionals may prescribe antiplatelet medications, such as aspirin, to reduce the risk of blood clots.

Regular Health Check-ups:

Regular Health Screenings:

Schedule regular health check-ups, including screenings for blood pressure, cholesterol, and blood sugar levels.

Medication Adherence:
Adhere to prescribed medications for hypertension, diabetes, and other conditions as directed by healthcare professionals.

Stroke Education and Awareness:

Know Family History:
Understand the family's medical history, especially regarding cardiovascular diseases and strokes.

Stay Informed:
Stay informed about stroke risk factors, symptoms, and preventive measures through healthcare professionals, reputable sources, and educational programs.

Prompt Medical Attention:

Understand the importance of seeking prompt medical attention if any signs or symptoms of a stroke are observed.

Regular Check-ups with Healthcare Professionals:
Establish a regular relationship with healthcare professionals for ongoing monitoring and preventive care.

By adopting a holistic approach that includes both lifestyle modifications and medical management, individuals can significantly reduce their risk of stroke. Regular communication with healthcare professionals and a proactive approach to managing risk factors are essential components of stroke prevention.

CONCLUSION

As we draw the curtains on this guide for stroke survivors and their caregivers, we want to underscore a message of resilience, hope, and unwavering support. The path to recovery after a stroke is undoubtedly challenging, but it is also a journey marked by profound courage and determination.

To the stroke survivors, you are not defined by the Challenges you face but by the strength with which you confront them. Each step forward, no matter how small, is a testament to your resilience. Embrace the victories, both big and small, and remember that your journey is unique, and healing unfolds at its own pace.

To the caregivers, your role is immeasurable. Your dedication, compassion, and patience create a foundation of support that enables your loved ones to face each day with newfound strength. Your tireless efforts do not go unnoticed, and your commitment is a source of inspiration for us all.

As we part ways, let us carry forward the lessons of adaptability, the importance of a strong support network, and the power of a positive mindset. The journey of stroke recovery is not one travelled alone; it is a collective effort, a shared narrative of triumph over adversity.

May this guide serve as a beacon of knowledge, encouragement, and understanding for both survivors and caregivers alike. Remember, beyond the Challenges lie opportunities for growth, moments of joy, and a future filled with possibilities.

Here's to the resilience within, the strength that binds us together, and the unwavering hope that lights our way. May your journey be marked by healing, love, and a brighter tomorrow."

Acknowledgement

I wish to acknowledge and heartily express my gratitude to the academic staff of the department of Internal Medicine and Surgery at the St. Thomas's Hospital, Michigan who mentored and provided the sound intellectual foundation and instrumental academic milieu for the success of this book. I want to especially recognize and applaud the efforts of the National Health Scheme, US/UK and the WHO, whose unwavering effort in the publication of statistics has aided the finished assembly of this book.

I wish to also acknowledge the immeasurable co-operation received from my Healthcare Provider.

I am grateful to Mr. Dominic Cyril who gave enormous secretarial assistance in the typing and formatting of the manuscript.

Disclaimer:

This book provides information and guidance intended for general educational purposes only. It is not a substitute for professional medical advice, diagnosis, or treatment. Readers should consult with a qualified healthcare professional for personalized recommendations regarding their specific condition. The author and publisher disclaim any liability arising directly or indirectly from the use of the information provided in this book. Individual responses to exercises, treatments, or lifestyle changes may vary, and readers should exercise caution and seek medical guidance before implementing any suggestions contained herein.